You Don't Need All That Makeup!!!

I0116848

By: Lianne Farbes

Foreword by: Jennifer Walsh

ISBN-13: 978-0615865348
ISBN-10: 0615865348:

DEDICATIONS

To My Mom & Dad – My teachers, protectors and defenders.. Mom - thank you for being my first beauty inspiration. The beautiful woman I got to see everyday that gave me new insight into all things. You taught me how to roll my hair, put on a face mask and bake bread. I love you both always and forever.

To My Son Tyler - Thank you for making me proud everyday. You always supported me even when times were tough. Mommy loves you.

To My Sister Stasi – Thank you for always making me laugh, supporting me, for letting me do your hair and makeup and for never complaining when I wanted you to be my guinea pig on a daily basis. I love you!

To Nana – Thank you for teaching me to be my own person, how to do reflexology, the importance of a face masque, how to drive, cut my own bangs, how to make a one egg cake and how to tie a scarf. I will love you always and will see you again one day.

To Grandmommie – Thank you for teaching me the beauty of a hot bath with bath oil, how to use Oil of Olay, and for some of my most popular sayings, "Waste not want not..." "Good Riddance to bad trash..", "Don't pay her any mind" and finally how to smile politely when you really don't want to. I love you and miss you.

To My OG Carrie - Thank you for always pushing, inspiring, loving, accepting and challenging me for more than 30 years. I love you!

To My Industry Greats - The Makeup Show, HBA Expo, BlogHer and anyone that has ever given me a platform to speak.....THANK YOU!! To all my beauty blogging sisters and all the beauty pioneers and editors that I have admired past and present...you inspire me!! To the makeup artists I have had the pleasure of meeting/working with and a few that I consider friends: Kevin James Bennett, James Vincent, Victoria Stiles, Viola Nicholson, Tia Dantzler, Billy B., Brian Duprey. I love you and thank you for providing such a wealth of information and for being such an inspiration to me on so many levels.

To My Readers – There would be no Makeup Girl without you. Thank you for allowing me to come into your home on a daily basis for 7 wonderful years. The best is yet to come!

FOREWORD BY: JENNIFER WALSH
FOUNDER OF THE BEAUTY BAR, PRIDE & GLORY BEAUTY
& BEHIND
THE BRAND MEDIA
NEW YORK, NY

If you have not had the chance to meet Lianne Farbes, here is your opportunity!

We girls in the beauty business usually stick together. We forge relationships and friendships that become a bond. Lianne and I have that kind of friendship. So when she approached me about writing this foreword for her book, I was so honored! For years I have watched as she continued to hone her craft through sheer determination and a true passion for the business. This book is the culmination of that passion.

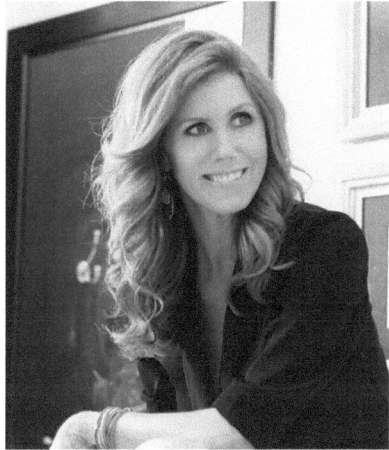

Lianne is not only a lover of all things beauty, but she is a true educator. Starting her blog back in 2006, she has worked diligently with brands directly to help them have a powerful voice within the world of beauty blogging.

This book is for anyone who wants great tips from a true beauty expert. You can almost hear Lianne and her insanely bubbly personality shine through the pages! She helps guide you through the beauty landscape of the true do's and don'ts and how to best use products at every stage of your life from your teenage years to maturity. "You Don't Need All That Makeup!!" is the essence of Lianne's career and of a woman who truly loves the beauty world.

Sit back and enjoy!

JENNIFER WALSH

YOU DON'T NEED ALL THAT MAKEUP!!!

INTRODUCTION

Hi, My name is Lianne and I am a beauty addict. Pleased to meet you! The only difference between you and me is experience. Why did I write this book? The reason, quite simply, is because I want to help YOU. There are many, MANY how to makeup and beauty guides out there, written by FABULOUS makeup artists and the like. What sets me apart? I have years of experience on multiple levels. I have been a model, makeup artist, makeup counter salesperson, makeup and skincare counter manager, and now on-air expert, blogger and sometimes makeup artist (again, but not really and only if my friends ply me with goodies and hugs). Over the past 20+ years, my experience has taken me to many different places, both personally and professionally.

There is nothing more I would like to do than help people achieve their personal beauty best whatever that may be. I love seeing the looks on their faces when they see a transformation! It is really a sight to behold, the confidence level rises and they feel like they can take on the world.

The business of beauty is very unique. It's the only industry that can elevate your mind, self-esteem and consciousness all at the same time. Have you ever seen someone after they leave the hair salon? They have a bounce in their step and confidence in their faces. That's what the power of beauty can do.

Speaking of the power of beauty.... I have seen it's power first hand, pretty much since the day I was born. The beauty bug had already bitten my mother and all my grandmothers. When I would visit my maternal grandmother (Nana) my sister and I would get to play dress-up in her clothes, scarves and jewelry. The big treat, however, was always getting to do facials with Queen Helene Mint Julep masque. When we visited my paternal grandmother (Grandmommie) in Nashville, it was all about reverse moon manicures, Oil of Olay and Jean Nate bubble baths. At home, my mother used Noxzema to take off her makeup and a moon drops peel off masque weekly. At Christmas I would get Tinkerbell makeup in my stocking. You know, the lipstick and sheer pink nail polish that peeled off!!?? I was obsessed. One day when I was 8 years old, I got to use REAL NAIL POLISH. I nearly died.

That night.... my sister and I painted our nails, ate appetizers of saltine crackers with deviled ham and watched the Sonny & Cher show. We marveled at Cher's Bob Mackie *fabulousness*. Later that year, someone (I don't remember who) took me to see Diana Ross in her new movie Mahogany after I did some serious begging. I was MESMERIZED. Her hair, her clothes, her makeup, her LASHES! That's the year when the beauty bug bit me.

If you have read my blog The Makeup Girl, you know that I am pretty much a straight shooter. I won't tell you something just because I think you want to hear it. Not every beauty product is for everybody. There is no one size fits all beauty. Just because it works for me doesn't mean it will work for you. Once you find a few looks that work for you...rock them until the wheels fall off. The best beauty (especially for everyday) is simplistic.

I want nothing more than to share my knowledge with you. I want for you to feel comfortable in your own skin. Beauty is more than makeup, it's about being the best YOU that you can be and that starts with great skin and a few tricks of the trade. This book is a basic guide for you to refer to whenever you need advice regarding anything beauty related.

So get out your highlighters and mark this book UP! Take notes and use it as your personal beauty guide. So sit back, relax and let me help you get there!

xoxo Lianne

CONTENTS

1 YOUR MOST IMPORTANT ASSET ✔

Your skin is most definitely your most important asset, without a doubt. Our skin is over 70% water and that being said, it needs constant attention like you would water a plant. Different outside factors affect our skin like weather, diet, pollution and alcohol. Its up to you to make sure you pay attention to your skin and give it what it needs so you can look your best. If you live in a severely cold climate, it's probably not a great idea to wear nothing to protect your skin.

Protection and maintenance are the hallmarks of great skin. Let's start with SPF. Everyone, regardless of how young or old you are should be wearing some kind of broad spectrum UVA/UVB Sun protection on a daily basis. That's just the way it is folks. Sunscreen is basically the fountain of youth. So if you want to look like you are 30 when your 40, put the baby oil down.

Now, I'm not saying you can't go to the beach or pool and have a good time. Of course you can. You just have to protect yourself when you do. The biggest mistake that women make is not using sun protection. I met a woman once that actually thought that SPF blocked the sun and would prevent her from getting a tan. I straightened her out...and if you think that then you need straightening out too. You will still tan, what you won't do is burn or contract skin cancer.

When it comes to your skin, your best defense is a good offense. You don't need to go crazy and spend hundreds of dollars but you do need to pay attention to ingredients and get yourself something that will help you achieve the look you want. I started using skincare religiously at 15 and haven't stopped since. It's kind of in my DNA. The women in my life taught me that taking care of my skin was important. When you are taught the importance of certain things at a young age, you stick with it. So it's important to establish routines.

I like to break mine up into things I do during the week. I only wash my hair once a week, so I do that on the weekend...usually Sunday. Matter of fact, *Sunday night beauty* is a ritual in my house. I usually do my hair during the day, put on a deep conditioner, and then at night, I'll do a mask and my nails (totally obsessed with nail stickers right now by the way). That's my routine...I started it LONG ago and it's just what I do.

During the week, I try and keep it minimal. I do mini scrubs in the shower...wash my face every day and night and slather on as many anti aging products as my skin can muster. When I traveled to Paris last year...looking at the women over there made me re-think how much makeup I wear for my daily routine. The women there have GLOWING skin, and you know what else? Red lipstick. That's it. Great skin and red lipstick. So now when I go out, I try to do only as much as I can get away with. Maybe some tinted moisturizer, mascara, bronzer and lips. I double up on my skincare.

Bottom line, take care of your skin and it will take care of YOU.

2 TAKE CARE OF YOUR SKIN ✔

Do you want skin so good you won't need makeup? It can be achieved but you have to be diligent. Do you take off your makeup every night? If not, you are setting yourself up for failure in the skin department. Leaving your makeup on while you sleep deprives your skin of much needed oxygen. There are even lazy girl ways to get it off if you don't feel like standing in front of the sink for 10 minutes. You can wear all the makeup in the world, but if your skin isn't in top shape then it doesn't matter what you put on it. It will also be painfully obvious that you are using the makeup to cover instead of enhance as the days go by. Hey, I like a Smokey eye just as much as the next gal, but at the end of the day, it's got to come off. The last thing we want is for your face to look like your wearing some kind of mask. We want your skin to look so good that you won't NEED makeup (you can wear it if you want to, but you won't need it). Let's start with taking OFF your makeup. Ready? Let's go.

Wash your hands first. So many people skip this step. It is probably the most important one. If you don't wash your hands before your touch your face, bacteria and outside elements are transferred to your skin. Bacteria causes breakouts...nuff said.

Remove your eye makeup. If you wear eye makeup, use a remover to ensure you get everything off. There are separate ones that work well for waterproof. Nana used Vaseline or Baby oil and a tissue...that works too.

Use a mild, gentle cleanser. Preferably one that also removes makeup. Always start on your forehead, and work your way down using circular motions. You can use a soap based or lotion based as long as it's mild. A cream based cleanser is a great for this because it takes everything off in one step.

Use a skincare tool. Not a vital step, but if you are into gadgets a sonic cleansing tool is fabulous at keeping your skin exfoliated and in top condition.

Rinse rinse rinse. Rinsing your face properly ensures you get any residue left behind.

Use a serum. Serums are like little skin specialists that help with specific issues. Like hyperpigmentation, dehydration, acne and even dry skin.

Layer your products appropriately. Always start with the thinnest in terms of consistency to the heaviest. We will touch more on this later.

3 SKINCARE 101 ✔

If you are still reading, then by now you SHOULD know all about my love for skincare. My earliest teen moment involved me and bottle of Ten-O-Six astringent. All my friends at school were using it, so I trotted off to Walgreens and bought a bottle. I got it home and marveled at how ORANGE it was.

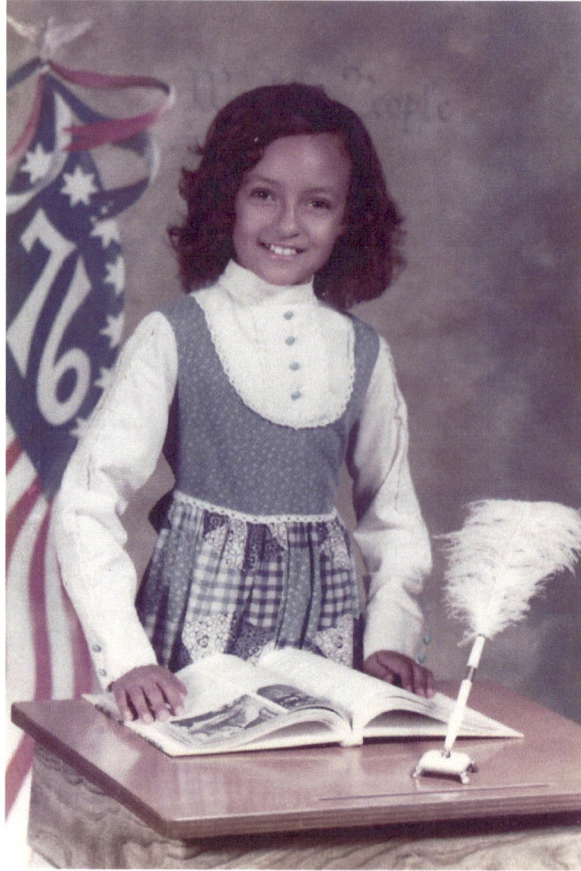

me in 4th grade

Most women these days talk to their daughters about skincare and makeup. But back then, we were pretty much winging it, with the help and advice of our friends, and Seventeen magazine. Turns out, Ten-O-Six (which looked like iodine by the way) was a bit too rough for my skin and my skin became overly dry. I learned through trial and error what worked for my skin and what absolutely didn't. So in order for you to do that, you need to SAMPLE. This is the perfect way for you to test things out before you try (which I love doing). I suggest getting some samples and testing things out to see how your skin reacts before you buy anything full size. You can even buy deluxe samples of EXPENSIVE products on eBay. Sampling can be a huge help before you buy.

Here are a few tips for sampling...

Visit Sephora. Sephora will ALWAYS give you samples of anything. So visit them and ask for Color IQ for makeup and Skincare IQ for skincare. They can use a computer to match your skin for foundation and the skincare IQ can scan barcodes with directions for use to go with the sample you receive.

Hit up GWP offers. Every department store has one. It's a great way to try before you buy if you need to pick up something else. SpaceNK stores have an event twice yearly where they have a big GWP. If you spend a certain amount you get a luxe gift bag filled with deluxe samples. You can use that one for a stock up session.

NOW...onto the skincare regimen.

Cleanser. This is all about personal preference as far as I am concerned. Some people like creamy cleansers, some prefer foam (I like both for different reasons). When choosing your cleanser, you have to take into account what you want your end result to be. These days, brands are making cleansers with all kinds of extras in them like retinol, fruit acid, brighteners etc. So if you have an issue you want to address, you can get some extra attention with your cleanser. The tried and true ones work just as good too, no need to spend a fortune.

Toner. While toners aren't a "must-have" part of *most people's* skincare regimen, they can be beneficial to your routine if you skin is particularly oily. I also like to use them in the summer as a refresher

Serum. A serum is like a moisturizer, but as I mentioned earlier it is really more like a skincare specialist. Serums have smaller molecules so they absorb a bit faster. You can add a serum to your routine to address a certain issue that maybe your moisturizer isn't able to help with. Look at it like a booster to your routine. Typical serums are anti-aging, firming, brightening...get the picture? You apply these BEFORE your moisturizer but after you cleanse/tone.

Moisturizer. No matter what, you need to add moisture to your skin. Like I said in the last section, even if you are oily you need to add hydration. The most common moisturizers are the humectant kind. No bells and whistles just a nice everyday moisturizer with an SPF. The next level contains some ingredients that you may or may not be familiar with. Take your time and ASK QUESTIONS. Especially when it comes to buying items at the department store. Many drugstores have associates that can help you with this as well.

Day Cream vs. Night Cream You really shouldn't be using a day cream with SPF at night. Why? Most moisturizers compromise their hydrating properties to accommodate the SPF. In addition, you don't want to leave an SPF on your skin while you sleep. Better to leave the SPF for the day as skin does the bulk of its repairing, restoring, and regenerating while we sleep, so night creams are focused on moisture and recovery.

Night Cream. Make sure that you are using an arsenal in the evening. Since this is when your body is in repair mode, you should be helping your skin to repair as well.

Layering. Make sure that you are applying your products from the thinnest to the thickest. This will ensure that your skin is getting what it needs the most FIRST. This is my order of operations for your face. After you wash your face and apply your toner (if needed) you should begin with the thinnest item you have (most likely this will be a serum or some other sort of booster). NOW.....If you have a booster or face oil then that goes first then next will come serum then the face cream. If you just have the serum - then that goes on first. Get it?

4 ACNE 101 ✔

Not everyone is blessed with flawless skin. For some people, it's genetics, but most have to work at it. During adolescence our skin is extremely hormonal causing all kinds of breakouts. Then our skin kind of relaxes until.... that's right it's coming. Middle age. Then the hormones go crazy again and your skin is ripe for more issues and breakouts. My skin is in THAT stage. Every month during "that time" I get breakouts on my chin (by the way, if you are getting breakouts on your chin it is always hormonal and definitely related to lady issues).

Follow these steps and your acne won't rule you.

Use products with active charcoal or sulfur. Activated charcoal which is a specially processed form of carbon has increasingly been used in many a beauty product. Charcoal, it's said, draws impurities and toxins out of the skin, helping to relieve acne and other skin problems. Sulfur is also a great way to treat breakouts, but it smells horrible. Kind of like a rotten egg, but hey who said beauty was painless?? Sulfur is one of the oldest known acne treatments. It's the same stuff match sticks are made of. Historically, it's known as brimstone (yes, *that* brimstone) and was used in ancient times to treat a multitude of skin issues such as warts, acne, dermatitis, dandruff and rosacea. Talk about multitasking!! Search for a product that is a scrub or a masque to treat your little problem. I have found that spot treatment with a sulfur mask for these little eruptions is quite effective.

Use heat. Do you ever get those horrible pimples that are underneath the surface? You know, the ones that hurt? I saw an esthetician back in my 20's that told me using a hot washcloth and massaging the pimple would help break it up and bring it to the surface. She was right and I still use that method to this day. It also makes it hurt less and takes the swelling down as well. I have also used a device called Zeno Hot Spot that does the trick as well.

Use salicylic acid. This ingredient was formerly only available by prescription. Now lower strengths are available over the counter. Start with the lowest strength you can find and apply once a day about half an hour after washing. Never use more than 5 percent strength without consulting a physician. It's a great option if your skin it too sensitive to tolerate a retinoid. Salicylic acid breaks up the layer of skin that clogs the sebaceous gland. This allows the pimple to heal and the pore return to normal.

Use retinoids. Topical retinoids come in three main classes and can be used to treat mild to medium cases of acne. Here is a listing of the most popular ones:

Adapalene is a synthetic retinoid used to unclog acne affected pores and may also be beneficial for reducing acne inflammation

Tazarotene works to unclog pores and reduce acne inflammation by increasing the turnover rate of skin cells on the acne affected areas of skin. Tazorotene has caused some birth defects in lab animals. Because of this, birth control is necessary at all times while you are using the topical medication.

Tretinoin is the only natural topical retinoid on the market and was also the first retinoid available for the treatment of acne. Like other retinoids, tretinoin works by promoting skin peeling and unclogging pores. Because of this, staying out of the sun and wearing SPF are essential to avoid unnecessary irritation.

Any of these will work fine; you can also find something called a micro retinoid that is available in some face creams. Doing your research or seeing a dermatologist is your best bet if you are uncertain.

Don't pick Whatever you do, it is very important to avoid scratching, popping or squeezing the pimples, this might lead to infection or scarring. Leave the extractions to the professionals.

Get regular facials Speaking of facials, treat yourself. Not only will this help the health of your skin (whether you have acne or not) but also they can do extractions for you if you have issues like blackheads. (I had one get out a blackhead that had been there so long; I thought it was a MOLE.) YIKES!

See a dermatologist If all else fails, you can make an appointment to see a dermatologist. They will be able to prescribe something topical or oral that you can take if over the counter methods aren't working.

5 ANTI-AGING 101 ✔

I'm 46 years old. There, I said it. I'll actually be 47 this year. I think age is all in how you carry and present yourself. I don't *feel* like I am approaching 50, but I am. That being said, I have worked hard over the years to take care of my skin. As a result, nobody believes me when I tell him or her my age. I still get carded sometimes which is ridiculous.... but it feels great. I will never turn down an opportunity to show my ID for anything age related.

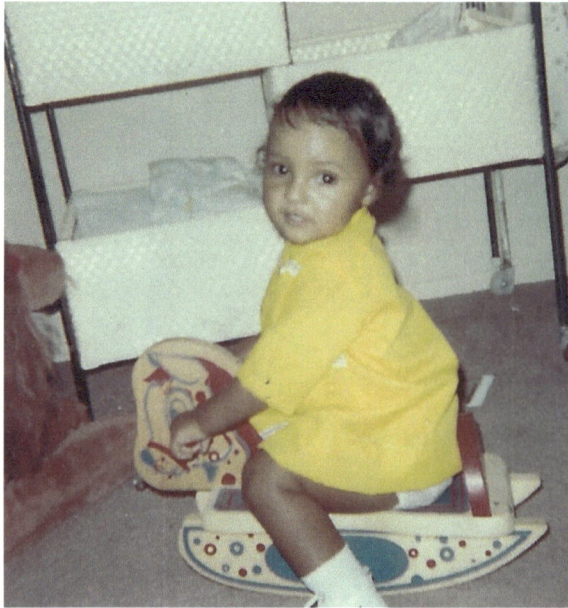

baby Lianne

My point is, don't be afraid of your age EMBRACE IT. If you don't like the way your skin looks, then DO SOMETHING ABOUT IT. This includes cosmeceuticals, injectables and whatever else you think is right, as long as it's done tastefully.

As far as skincare is concerned, the best way to approach anti-aging is to add products to your routine. Maybe you didn't exfoliate when you were younger, now you may need to. Listen to your skin and make adjustments accordingly. When to start? I would say your late 20's you should be thinking about it. Early 30's are a good time to start. If you are a teenager, you can start with SPF and a good regimen of taking care of your skin on a daily basis, your 40 year old face will thank you later.

Taking care of things takes discipline; it's just like anything else. People don't get ripped bodies just by sitting around. The same is true for your skin. You have to WORK at it. Here are a few tips to get you started on your road to skincare discipline.

Step up your moisturizer in your 30's. Now is the time to add a moisturizer with a little more muscle. Look for anti-aging ingredients like resveratrol, retinol and micro-retinol in addition to whatever new ingredients that are out on the market. Do your research, speak to professionals, get some samples and explore. If you are past your 30's, then start adding serums and boosters (its never too late!). It's also a good idea to see a dermatologist or a facialist and start regular treatments.

Exfoliate. Exfoliation removes the top layers of the skin, which have built up as skin cell turnover slows down with aging. By removing the outer layers, you reveal younger newer layers underneath and help the skin to increase cell turnover. Be careful with the exfoliation though, it can make your skin sensitive to the sun (chemical exfoliators are the culprit here). You can also use a good old-fashioned washcloth or a sonic cleansing brush. If you are in doubt about any of these methods, pay a visit to your dermatologist.

Treat. There are a certain number of ingredients that appear in most clinical studies that get the job done. As far as anti-aging goes, those are peptides, anti-oxidants, retinoids and SPF. I also pay attention to anything new coming down the pike that is billed as the newest anti-aging wonder (you should too!) I know I have mentioned SPF a few too many times in this book, but do you know why? Ask any dermatologist and they will tell you that wearing SPF is the single most effective way to combat aging. Plus it's the fountain of youth (I said that already, didn't I??)

Quit Smoking. You shouldn't be doing this anymore. So if you are, you should know that in addition to casing bad breath and cancer, it also destroys collagen, elastin and decreases estrogen levels.

Stay Hydrated. I'm not talking about just drinking water (which you should be doing anyway so put down the diet coke please). You can use a humidifier at night that will help keep skin moist. I also like using a HOT moist face cloth when I take off my makeup. Any way to increase hydration is good in my book.

Get Some Sleep. I am guilty of this one on more than a regular basis. Your skin requires downtime to repair itself and existing on no sleep will do nothing to decrease sagging or puffiness around the eyes.

6 SAFETY 101 ✔

I get so many emails asking about the shelf life of skincare and makeup. I had one reader say that she had the same face cream from 2009!! Not pretty ladies. Just like cosmetics, skincare has a shelf life especially after it has been opened. So how are you supposed to know when to toss things out? European companies have used the PAO (Period After Opening) or "**Open Jar Symbol**" for quite some time now.

Now this symbol is starting to catch on in the states, which is a good thing. Take a look on the back of your skincare, there will be an open jar with a number and "m" next to it. That tells you how long the item is good after it has been opened. For instance "12m" means 12 months.

In the past, this symbol was almost exclusively used for skincare but now it is being included on some makeup. When you buy a product, put a little round sticker on it with the month/date on it when you open it. That way you can keep track of when you bought it.

Here is a guide to follow...

Skincare

Preface this by saying, if you are using it like you are supposed to, they should be gone within 12 months.

Face cream. 12-14 months no question. Try not to use your fingers to avoid contamination (make sure your fingers are clean). You can always use the spatula that comes with the jar as well.

Organics. If the item in question is organic or has plant based ingredients, the shelf life is much shorter. There is a higher chance of contamination because they don't use traditional methods of preserving so I would say 1 year at the MOST.

Face Wash. 12 months but again it really should be lasting you a shorter period of time unless you buy an industrial size!

Eye Cream. 12 months. Because it is a product that is near your eyes, there is a higher risk of contamination.

Makeup

Makeup is a bit trickier because they have different ingredients. Here is a guide....

Concealer. These will last up to 12 months depending on the formula. Cream based ones last a bit longer.

Powder. Up to 2 years.

Pencil eye liner. These should be sharpened regularly and can last up to 3 years.

Eyeshadow. These can last up to 3 years although you will hit the pan on them far before that if you use them regularly.

Foundation. Check the ingredients: A water-based foundation will last up to 12 months, oil-based will last up to 18 months.

Lip liner. These can last up to 3 years.

Lipstick. 1-2 years, BUT the best way to tell is, if it smells rancid or funny, toss it.

Mascara. 2-3 months. Keep a close eye on these because if they aren't closed tightly, they can dry out faster.

Nail Polish. Up to 12 months, depending on the quality.

Tools

Brushes. Wash every month in a mild detergent. (More on that later.)

Sponges. Wash weekly and discard monthly. Unless it is a beauty blender sponge. These sponges have specific requirements for cleansing and shelf life.

Bottom line, if it smells funny – TOSS IT. My last tip is always, always, ALWAYS wash your hands BEFORE you touch your products or your face. If you are touching your products with unwashed hands you are contaminating them – plain and simple. Think of it this way, whatever you touched that day is going into the product and onto your face.... not pretty. So check your products and be safe!

7 MAKEUP 101 ✔

Now that you have FLAWLESS skin, it's time to put on a little makeup. Some of you will like this chapter more than others but ultimately, the look we are going for is the most beautiful and enhanced version of you. This is especially important for those of you that don't normally wear makeup. You don't want to look like a different person...just enhanced. We are stocking your makeup bag! I am a big fan of brands that make shades that match a wide range of skin tones.

When I started modeling as a teenager, there were NO foundations that matched my skin (and I mean NONE). If you look at some of the ads I appeared in, my face looks ghastly and gray like a ghost.

One day, the makeup artist on one of my jobs was changed and so was my life. He taught me how to take Joe Blasco cream and make my own shade. I was never without a color again. Picking a foundation has to be one of the hardest things to do.

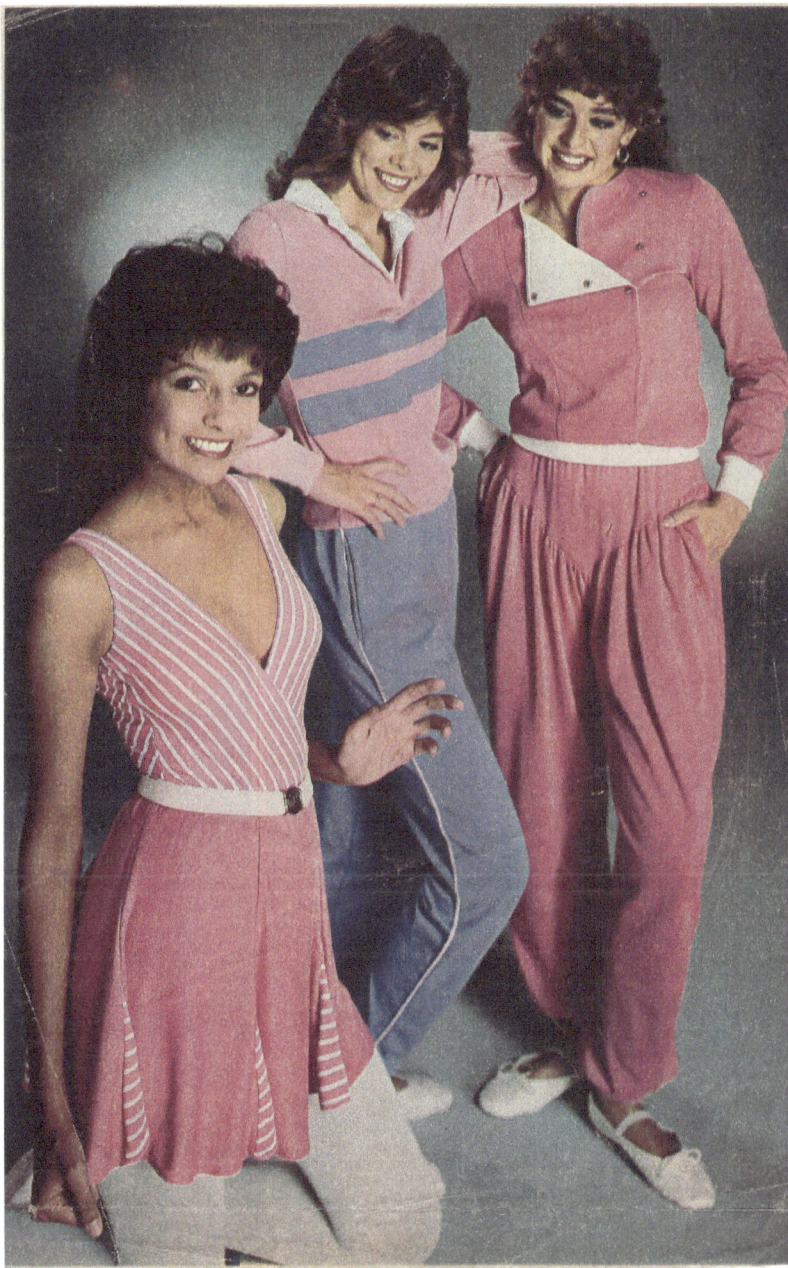

Old Modeling pic from the 80's GRAY GHOST FACE!!

Most women can't find a shade to match and even if you do – you still may be between two shades. Then there is the dreaded counter salesperson. I actually had someone recently try to sell me a shade that was CLEARLY darker than my skin.

So the more information you are armed with when you shop, the better. Make sure they are testing the shade on your jawline (something I learned when I was a custom blender for the now defunct Prescriptives). The shade that disappears into your skin is the one for you. Sometimes that means two...sometimes people need to do a little mixing. If this is you, I suggest you go see someone that is a makeup artist. Not everyone that works at Sephora and the department store is a makeup artist, nor are they all well versed with custom blending. I have a few tips for you to get you started.

Use social media. Pay attention to Instagram, Twitter and Facebook. Most makeup artists are on any one of these social platforms (sometimes all three) and are happy to answer questions when they have the time.

Research brands. Find a brand that speaks to your lifestyle, not all of the best brands can be found in the department store/drugstore. Sometimes you have to go off the beaten path.

Attend Consumer events. There is an event called The Makeup Show, which is in several US cities, as well as a few in Europe. You can get face to face with makeup artists, brands and ask questions.

You can also get a pretty sweet discount too!

Now...onto application. Here is my guide for a pretty flawless face with minimal effort.

Foundation. I don't even really like that word. BUT, I understand its necessity. I am a big fan of natural looking product that looks like skin and not a mask. But that is about application more than anything. Select a product that will give you the coverage you are looking for and invest in a good makeup brush. You will use this to blend. Hourglass Cosmetics has a full coverage foundation in two formulas (one for oily skin called Immaculate and one for normal to dry skin called Veil). Both of these give full coverage BUT feel like your skin, which I am a huge fan of. I even like the newer BB and CC creams out there because they give you good coverage with a lightweight feel. I also like to use a baked powder with some luminosity to dust all over on top for finishing.

Cheeks. Cream to powder ones last a bit longer in my opinion. For this, I like to use a multi-use stick that you can place on your cheeks, nose, and lips. The goal is to look kind of like you were in the sun.

Eyes. For a natural everyday look, I like to use a creamy product, simply because I like to put something on at the beginning of the day and not worry about it. I use Clinique *Chubby Sticks* and *Quickliner* practically on a daily basis. They are inexpensive and EASY to use.

Eyebrows. No mater whether your are a blonde or brunette filling in your brows is essential as brows frame your face. I would suggest a pencil that has a bit of wax in it to offer more control. For grooming, I would make an appointment to get your brows threaded, waxed or if you are handy with the tweezers. Whatever you do, keep them groomed. Eyebrows are like the frame for your face.

Lips. This is more about preference than anything. If you like lipstick then feel free to experiment with different colors. If you prefer something more lightweight, you can go with a gloss. Application is important here too, use a brush or your fingers instead of taking it straight from the tube, your product will last longer and you will get more precise application.

8 CONCEALER 101 ✔

We don't need you running around town looking like a raccoon now do we? Are you over 30 or fast approaching? If so, please take my advice and start using a concealer. It really does make a world of difference *when applied correctly*. When I say correctly, I mean **use a brush** and DAB. That way you can **control** the amount of product so you can avoid the cakey look. In addition, if you have puffiness problems see my hangover chapter for a DIY remedy with a certain household item!

Application. When applying your concealer, the first and most important thing is your brush. You need a small brush that can be easily controlled. I recommend Bobbi Brown's concealer brush or Bare Essentials concealer brush. Both brushes are super easy to handle and because of their small size, you never risk getting too much product on the brush itself, eliminating the whole cakey thing.

Now for color. When choosing a concealer, you want to make sure it counteracts the blue-ish area under your eyes. Always get one that has a bit of peach in it. If you use a concealer the same color as your foundation it will only *accentuate the circles* and make them look even more pronounced. The peachy tone will counteract the gray tones flawlessly. Select a creamier formula for the delicate area under your eye so you don't have to do any tugging. For other areas, you can go with a drier formula. For under eye application, **DAB** the concealer under your eye and brush outward. You can use the brush to blend as well. Just make certain that the edges disappear into your skin. You want to make certain that the edges of the concealer vanish into your skin so blending is essential here.

When concealing other areas such as a blemish or a birthmark, DAB the concealer on the object to conceal and blend the edges. Be careful though, if you put too much product on, you will end up drawing more attention to the issue. Concealer adheres best to clean dry skin so make certain that its the first thing that you do, then follow with your foundation and powder. If you are using a full coverage foundation – you can put that on first then get any areas that the foundation doesn't reach with the concealer on top.

Here are a few of my favorites...

Eve Pearl Salmon Concealer. If you have dark circles, this is the one for you. This amazing peachy color neutralizes the dark blue undertones from the skin. (Yellows mixed with the blue undertones create those greenish/grey raccoon eyes that are highlighted and only accentuate the problem area.) This is a creamy formula that blends effortlessly.

Bobbi Brown Creamy Concealer. Great consistency and color. Comes in a cute little flip top container with a mirror. Perfect for everyday and works on blemishes, age spots and other dark marks.

MAC Studio Finish Concealer. Is a lightweight and creamy opaque concealer. It also comes in great shades and will cover ANYTHING. I have used it to cover a black eye and a tattoo! It also contains SPF 35.

BECCA Compact Concealer. This is a true favorite of mine because the color range is AMAZING! This mini compact has two concealers. On one side there is a heavier more opaque formula and on the other a sheerer one. You can mix and match to get the coverage you need.

9 SPF 101 ✔

I have been using sunscreen regularly since I was 9 or 10. We grew up in Southern California and had a pool. My sister and I spent a lot of time out there, swimming and running around. One day my mother had to run an errand or something. So for whatever reason she was gone for the afternoon. Guess who was in charge? Yep, Dad. So of course my sister and I begged to get in the pool, and of course he said yes. We jumped in - and we stayed out there ALL DAY. We played, we swam, and we ate hot dogs. Then later on, mom gets home and practically screams that we had been burned. In our haste, we had on no sunscreen (dad didn't put any on us and we forgot). We were out in the sun between 11 and 3. I had a black and white striped one-piece swimsuit on and when I took it off, I was striped because the suit wasn't lined. Needless to say, Dad wasn't left in charge all that much going forward! As I stated in an earlier chapter, SPF is the fountain of youth so bottom line, SPF is important and is **necessary** to maintain your youthful appearance.

Let me break it down for you...

How does it work? A sunscreen with a minimal SPF of 15 filters approximately 92% of the UVB rays. What does that mean? Basically a sunscreen with an SPF of 15 will delay the onset of sunburn in a person who would otherwise burn in 10 minutes to burn in 150 minutes. The SPF 15 sunscreen allows a person to stay out in the sun 15 times longer. Sunscreen actually filters the suns rays and ALLOWS you to stay in the sun longer without burning.

If you are in doubt, see a dermatologist who can give you a plethora of information on how damaging the sun can be to your skin if left unprotected.

Figure it out. Multiply the number of the SPF by how long you are staying in the sun. Example: SPF 15 x 20 minutes of sun time = 300. This is how many minutes you can stay in the sun without burning. So 300 minutes divided by 1 hour of 60 minutes = 5 hours of sun protection without a sunburn.

Use a minimum sunscreen daily. You should use a minimum of 15, but no more than 50-70 (anything higher than this is unnecessary). Re-apply often, especially if you are going in the water. My arms and hands always get hit the hardest because I do a lot of driving. The windshield magnifies the sun so I use a hand cream with sunscreen and applies it often.

Outdoors. If you are planning to be outdoors in any capacity, you need a sunscreen. This means, hiking, running, sunning, swimming, working out or basically ANYTHING. I am particularly fond of the new formulas you can just spray on. I leave it by my door on the way out to spray my arms so I don't forget.

Kids. Children need sunscreen too! If they squirm, spray them, if they complain, spray them. Spray...spray...SPRAY! Better yet, if they see YOU putting it on, they will too. Lead by example.

10 SELF TANNER 101 ✔

Self-tanners are a FABULOUS way to fake a tan and get a little bit of a glow on winter weary skin. They are also a great alternative to actual sunbathing as well. Experiment with different brands and understand that you don't have to spend a fortune to get one that will do the trick.

The first time I used a self-tanner was a lifetime ago when I was living in Los Angeles. Back then; they only had one color (there was no light to medium or medium to dark). It just wasn't that sophisticated. I had a friend that would use self tanner and just walk around nude until it dried. That would require too much work for me and plus I *am 100% too impatient* for that. I applied some to my arms and legs and I waited. I saw no results in the allotted time so of course I applied more (I'm impatient!). I ended up looking like an Oompa Loompa and got it all over my clothes. It took me a week to get back to normal. Thank goodness for technology! Things like that rarely happen these days! I even like to use the gradual moisturizing products like *Jergens Natural Glow* to get my skin out of the winter doldrums in the spring. It just kind of wakes everything up.

If you have never used a self tanner before, there is a bit of a learning curve but nothing you can't handle! Here are a few pointers...

Do a patch test. I know...I know but you could be sensitive to certain ingredients in the product. Better to be safe than sorry! Test the product on the inside of your wrist to see how the tone looks and to be sure you don't have a reaction. You can always return it if you have issues.

Remove hair in advance. If you use depilatory or you are a waxer wait 24 hrs. If you shave wait 12 hrs.

Exfoliate. You will get better results if you do this ahead of time. Get rid of all the dead skin so you can start fresh. Use a scrub or a mud mask 24 hours ahead of time.

Use gloves. Protect your hands from stains by using a pair of rubber gloves. Not the kind you wash dishes, but the kind you can get at your drugstore in the medicine aisle. Many self-tanners these come with gloves too.

Stay out of the water. No swimming, bathing or sweating for at least 8 hours. So stay out of the gym and skip your shower. You don't want all your hard work going down the drain right?

What if your color is wrong or streaky? No problem! There are several ways you can get back to square one.

Baking soda paste. You can make a paste with baking soda and water and rub the affected area (this works really great on your face). Work in a circular motion, rinse and repeat.

Hop in the water. If the area is more widespread, you can start over by hopping in the pool (the chlorine will help speed up the process) or take a nice long bath with a little scrub mitt and get to work!

11 FALSE EYELASHES 101 ✔

Don't be scared of false lashes! You can get a little extra glamour by yourself! The thing people seem to be most afraid of when it comes to applying the lashes themselves is that they think it will be difficult. This is a HUGE misconception because I think they are super easy to apply. The biggest mistake people make is the size or style of lash. You don't want them to look fake. You just want to look like you have more fullness and volume. The goal is not to have lashes that look like a doll from the 1940's but look like luxuriously long fluttery lashes that grew out of your eyes.

Choose a style. I prefer Ardell Wispy, MAC No 7 Lash or Shu Uemura's Soft Cross. Either of these will give you the drama you are looking for without looking fake.

Adhesive. Make sure you get glue that is black or clear and not white. If you can only find white make sure the tube says dries clear.

Mascara. Put your mascara on FIRST. NEVER put mascara on top of false lashes, it lessens their longevity. Use lengthening/defining mascara. Apply at least 2 coats if not three waiting 1 minute in between to ensure that each coat is dry before you put on the next. This will cut down on clumps.

Application. Take a toothpick (if you have an old pair of tweezers, you can use those too) squeeze a small amount of glue from the tube and dip it in. Then...

- Hold your lash seam side up.

- Drag the toothpick along the seam of the lash applying a thin layer of glue.

- Holding your eye at half-mast (or looking down into a mirror) take the lash and hold it as close to the lash line as possible.

At this point, you have about a minute before the glue dries so make adjustments accordingly and when you get them where you want them, then leave them alone for at least 5 minutes so the glue can set. Pinch the lash and your lash together.

Voilà now you have high drama lashes! Honestly, it is not as hard as it looks. Why not pick up a pair and play with them? You will get the hang of it I promise!

12 LIQUID EYELINER 101 ✔

The newest trend these days is liquid liner. Now I know what you are thinking, "*No way am I gonna wear that 60's batwing liner like Amy Winehouse!*" You don't have to, unless you want to that is! Liquid eyeliner has gotten a bad rap through the years. You actually can wear it and make it subtle – even for everyday.

If you like black then GO FOR IT. I mean it, go all out. If you think black is too harsh for you, the best way to keep it soft is to use a color *that's right.... color*. Go for a soft brown or even one of the new fun metallic versions. I also love the newer gel cream liners you can use with a brush. There are also alternatives to the standard brush method like the liner pen. I really like Lancôme Artliner. It comes in great colors and it is pretty foolproof, it's just a little marker pen.

Whatever you do, don't be afraid of it, fear is your worst enemy here. Relax and keep a pointed cotton swab and some eye makeup remover nearby just in case. But if you follow my tips, you won't need them.

Keep your eyes open. With your head tilted slightly back (keeping your eyes closed while applying can be disastrous.) Keeping your eye open will allow you to follow the natural contour of your eye. You can also lift your lid a bit and get right into the lash line without a gap.

Start at the inner corner of your eye. Make little dashes all the way across your lash line and then connect them. This way you can build on it if you think the look is too subtle. If you want a little wing on the end, start small and build.

Keep your shadow soft. If you use a soft shadow in a neutral tone, it will ensure that the focus is on the cat eye line and not the shadow.

Keep your stroke fast. This makes it is much easier to get the line done. Use short quick strokes rather than spend 15 minutes agonizing over it. As long as you stay close to the lash line, you can always go back.

Keep the tail short. I don't really love the elongated tail it looks so exaggerated, but if you must keep it short and extend only a teeny bit beyond the end of your eye. You can add more to the tail after the initial line is in the can.

Here are a few more brands I love....

MAC Fluidline. You will need to buy a MAC 209 brush (or something similar) and have a steady hand for this one, but practice makes perfect. These come in an array of great colors and the formula is a gel crème so it is very easy to work with.

Clinique Eye Defining Liquid Liner. This only comes in two shades (black and brown) but the great fast drying formula makes this a good standby to have in your bag.

Bobbi Brown Longwear Gel Liner. This is also one of my favorites. It calls for a steady hand like the MAC liner, but the colors and the formula are amazing.

13 SMOKEY EYE 101 ✔

It was 2011, and MAC Cosmetics had contacted me about a top-secret project they were working on. A capsule collection designed entirely by BLOGGERS. AMAZING! So wonderful to have been thought of in the first place, and with 100 others also in the running I thought maybe I had a shot.... maybe not? Oh who was I kidding!! I was CRAZY with nerves.

So, we had to do a presentation of sorts to show our chosen shade and the inspiration behind it. I prepared my required digital presentation, chose a name, answered my questions...closed my eyes and hit send. Then I promised myself I would let it go. I had done my best and if this didn't work out, there would surely be other opportunities like this one (there haven't been any by the way).

Then one day months later, I got a phone call out of the blue from Erin McCaffrey who was a Vice President at MAC at the time. She said, "Hi Lianne, its Erin from MAC." I was silent for a few seconds (Why was Erin calling me on my cell phone??!!) then I said, "Hey Erin...so nice to hear from you." Then I kind of don't remember the rest all that well (I blacked out...it was a blur...something about congratulations.... you need to have your passport...blah blah...we will be leaving for Toronto in a few weeks...blah blah blah). I'm pretty sure I told her to shut up a few times and threw in a NO WAY?! and Are you SERIOUS??! She was serious and before I knew it I was crying and my mother thought something was wrong.

It was such an overwhelming feeling that I can't really describe to you. My friend Patrice Grell Yursik (who was also one of the bloggers chosen for her "All of my Purple Life" lipglass concept) said it best when we were talking about it.

She said, "*It's something that I didn't realize that I wanted for myself, until it was actually happening.*" She hit the nail on the head.

NO ONE <3'S M·A·C BLOGGERS' OBSESSIONS MORE THAN YOU! BY POPULAR DEMAND, SOLD-OUT SHADES OF EYE SHADOW AND LIPGLASS BY BEAUTY BLOGGING SUPERSTARS AMBER, WENDY, AILEEN, LIANNE, CHRISTINE, PATRICE, LILY, KAREN AND LESLEY ARE BACK. FEED YOUR OBSESSION TODAY! AVAILABLE EXCLUSIVELY ONLINE.

SHOP NOW

I was SO EXCITED to have been chosen for the opportunity to be included in the MAC Cosmetics Bloggers Obsessions collection. I knew immediately that I wanted to do a shadow for a smokey eye. It's the one thing that I think people have trouble doing. My shade was called **Hocus Pocus** (the original name was *Smokin' In The Girls Room* but it didn't pass the legal department). It sold out TWICE, and it has long since been discontinued (I have a stock pile because I bought them, all up when they were in the goodbye section on the MAC website!) You can find it on eBay or maybe on some swap sites if you are interested. I wish you could have one! There are so many bad versions of this timeless look floating around.

A good smokey eye says glamour, but a BAD one says so much more. Don't go for the dark black shadows you see on the runway and in the magazines if you don't know what you are doing (and in some cases, even if you do!) It most always comes out looking muddy, unprofessional and quite frankly like you got punched in the eye (dirty makeup brushes are the likely culprit here). So we don't want that!! Stick to shades that are in the grey, deep brown, plum and even green families. They are easier to work with, and will look subtle as opposed to your eye-makeup being the first thing people notice. You want them to notice your EYES and THEN your makeup.

Here are a few tips that I have picked up over the years:

Use a good base. ALWAYS use a shadow base in a shade closest to or a bit darker than your eyelid. I have found that the primers that have a lot of shimmer in them tend to **change the colors of the shadow** and can come off looking quite garish – steer clear. I like to use MAC Paint Pots, and with a CLEAN fibre brush. Place this on your eyelid (but not the brow bone). The shadow/look will last much longer when it has something to adhere to.

Shadow. Choose a shadow that compliments your eye color. Use CLEAN brushes. If your brushes are NOT clean it can contribute to the muddy look I spoke of above. Another thing you want to make sure of is that you use a HIGHLY pigmented shadow. If you use a shadow that doesn't have enough pigment, not only will the look not last, it will end up looking more natural than anything else. You can test the pigmentation of shadows in the store. Take a shadow applicator and sweep it across the product, test a bit on your hand if it shows up after ONE sweep, the pigmentation is high. If it takes several sweeps then move on.

Placement. Place the shadow closest to your lash line to start. You can even lift your brow a bit to get the area right near the lash line that often get's missed. Then, with a blending brush, blend upwards towards your brow bone. You can add another color in a lighter shade on your brow bone, but the blending is imperative in order for it to look seamless. Remember, your eyes don't have to be dark like coal in order for it to qualify as a smokey eye. It just needs to have a shade that is noticeably darker than your eye color.

Fallout. This is when your shadow ends up under your eyes after you apply it. The best way to counteract this is to do your eyes first, clean up with some eye makeup remover and then apply your foundation. They also make shields that sit under your eyes, but a tissue also works very well. Fallout varies from brand to brand so make sure you cover your bases.

Here are some of my favorites:

NARS Cordura Shadow Duo. This is my go to shadow for a foolproof brown/bronzey look. This with a little Smolder Pencil from MAC and you has smokey eye heaven.

Bobbi Brown Eyeshadow in Caviar. When I want something a little deeper, I reach for this. The Caviar shade is magical but you can make your own palette with whatever shades you want! If Caviar is too deep for you, then go for a nice matte brown.

Urban Decay Naked Palette. This is a great starting point for a foolproof selection of blendable, coordinated smokey eye choices. However, most may find the large selection of choices a bit overwhelming.

No matter what shadows you use, make sure you take your time. Smokey eyes can look fantastic or horrific. Make sure yours are on the fantastic side. Watch some YouTube videos and educate yourself. You will be a master in no time!

14 BRONZER 101 ✔

Having a little color year round is okay; you just have to make sure that you switch your colors out for fall and winter. Otherwise you will end up looking a gilded mess. The use of bronzer is a great way to wake up your skin; I prefer colors that are matte and not glittery (a little shimmer is okay just not GLITTER). Some of my favorite bronzers actually have little or no glitter in them at all, and some of the newer ones that are baked are really great. Make certain that you have a good brush specifically for your bronzer. Sephora has a great one that is domed and easy to use.

I also love to have a pop of pink on my cheeks in addition to the bronzer, it ensures a radiant glow. Place the pink shade on first where the sun hits your face (forehead, nose, chin and apples of your cheeks). Apply your bronzer right under the apples of your cheeks and sweep outward.

My Nana bought me my first bronzer from Saks when I was 16 (it was Guerlain Terra Cotta.... those tortoise shell compacts are DIVINE) and I have been hooked ever since. Contrary to popular belief, bronzer can be worn YEAR ROUND. I have even been known to mix a bronzer cream or gel in with my moisturizer in the winter just so I can get that glow.

Here are some of my favorites:

Laura Geller Bronze-n-Brighten The baked formula is great, and the colors have no orange which ensures it is very flattering on any skin tone.

NARS The Multiple Bronzer This is my absolute favorite one stop shopping multi-use stick. The cream to powder formula can be used on eyes cheeks or body. It gives a warm pretty glow, it is super easy to work with and they have no shimmer at all.

Geurlain Terra Cotta The original bronzing powder for the soft sun kissed look now comes in *8 shades* so you can use one for summer and another for winter.

Bobbi Brown Matte Bronzer This lovely compact comes in 6 shades that will give you your PERFECT matte bronze look with zero shimmer.

Hard Candy So Baked Bronzer This is by far the least expensive option, but probably one of the BADDEST. Hard candy has somehow managed to get a baked matte bronzer with a teeny but of shimmer into a $9 package.

15 HANGOVER 101 ✔

Weddings, the holidays, birthdays. Life is just party after party, with way too much wine and champagne and far too little food. So it's safe to say that many a *diva* no matter what walk of life you come from has come home from an evening out on the town tired. Please don't sleep in your makeup! Not only will you be doing your skin a disservice, but your lovely bed linens as well. I have a plan that your skin and eyes will love. They will also thank you in the morning, when you are in the midst of your hangover.

When we go out, there are a number of circumstances that are beyond our control. Atmosphere is one of them. Also, when we drink (no matter how much or how little we consume), we get dehydrated. Dehydration means that our skin gets dehydrated too! Follow a few simple steps before you crash and a few more in the morning, and your skin will thank you.

Wash your face. I know that many of us will not feel like actually washing our faces. That's why I have another solution that will get your face clean and not dry it out. If you don't feel like actually washing your face, get over to Target and pick up some makeup remover towelettes. I like Yes To Blueberries Brightening Wipes. They have a great package with a little door so they won't dry out (I hate it when that happens). They will get everything off even eye-makeup and mascara, even if you are a little tipsy.

Use a good moisturizer. Remember what I said about dehydration? Well it goes double for your skin after a night on the town. Make sure you slather on the night cream. For the super lazy, you can even keep a sample of your favorite and makeup remover wipes in your bedside drawer within easy reach.

Drink plenty of water. Or some other kind of hydrating beverage. I shouldn't have to tell you this, but if you are in the dark then let me enlighten you. For every drink you consume, you should have one glass of water (it works). In addition, hydrate yourself frequently the day after your night on the town. Drinking on an empty stomach is also a big no-no. Have *something* to eat first.

Take some Emergen-C. This wondrous powder is 1000mg of Vitamin C and electrolytes (we lose those when drinking too!) all in a little packet. Sprinkle it in 4oz of water before you go to sleep or the morning after. You will feel much, much better.

Keep teaspoons in your freezer. I know it sounds weird, but hear me out. A makeup artist back in the day taught me this trick. Place two teaspoons in the freezer and use them on your eyes for puffiness. Lie down, and hold them on your eyes for at least 5 minutes. Better than any tea bag! Now don't ask me which side of the spoon to use, you will figure it out on your own. I even went and bought some a la carte spoons at Target, so now I have my freezer spoons.

Stick your face in an ice bath. Remember, ice reduces swelling. So if your face is swollen, you can fill a bowl with water and two trays of ice and immerse your face. The swelling will be sent packing. I know it sounds terrifying but whoever said beauty was easy???

If you follow these steps, I guarantee you, your skin will be soft, refreshed, tight and toned. After you have taken care of your skin, make sure you go out for a huge breakfast (preferably with hash browns, eggs and some kind of sausage or bacon) the next day.

16 TRAVEL 101 ✔

I am a reformed, disorganized over packer. In the fall of 2012, I went to Paris for a few days of beauty and cultural adventure. Guess what? I was CARRY ON ALL THE WAY! Did you hear me? I used a carry on when I flew to Paris!! I didn't check one thing except for all the beauty products I bought in a separate bag on the way back!

The last time I was in Paris was December 2000. If I recall correctly, I threw everything into a giant rolling duffle bag and got on the plane. Not pretty. But back then pre 9/11, travel was EASY. There was NO security, and you could take anything on the plane you wanted (even a corkscrew). It was pretty much the easiest trip I had ever taken. These days, there is SO much to worry about. What you can and can't take, should I carry on, what can I pack, what CAN'T I pack.

I used to put everything into a suitcase and end up wearing 5 things. Or I would take full sized beauty items in a big zippered bag. So when my expert traveler friend Julia Coney saw me in New York September of 2012. Her jaw dropped. She took one look at the bag I packed for 4 days and said with a straight face, *"You can't pack like this when we go to Paris Lianne."*

She knew I didn't wear half the things in my suitcase. Turns out I had what I thought was a pair of boots...yeah it was one left and one right from different pairs. I didn't use half the products I brought with me either.

So she helped me devise a plan to get organized.

Here it is in a condensed format....

Make lists. Julia turned me on to the *Evernote app* to keep me organized. I started clipping things off the web I wanted to save and I made lists. I even made a *packing list* so I knew what I was bringing and I mapped out outfits.

Carry on. Especially if you are Staying 10 days or less. You save money on baggage fees AND you don't have to stress about your luggage getting lost. I have a 20-inch Swissgear carry on approved suitcase. It was $89 at Target. They also have a nice one now that has a padded laptop pocket too.

Organize your clothes. I used a SpacePak from Flight001. My friend Felicia Walker Benson turned me on to this one when we went to LA a few years back. See!!! I've been trying to be a good packer, and I just relapse repeatedly. The SpacePak is brilliant, because it forces you to fit everything into that little zippered space (no overpacking). Plus, there is a spot on the other side for dirty clothes.

Pack an extra bag. If you know you are going to do some shopping, pack a duffle and check THAT on the way back. I have one from LeSportSac that I was able to fold up and put in the bottom of my carry on.

When in doubt, compartmentalize. Julia is big on pouches and I can't say that I blame her. I like having things all together because then I know exactly where they are. There is nothing worse than arriving at your destination and realizing you don't have the charger for your laptop or smartphone. For international travel, you have to make sure you have your passport for EVERYTHING so I got this GREAT padded pouch from Otis Batterbee where I stashed my wallet, passport and phone.

Makeup. I have a love/hate relationship with this tip. Even though I pretty much wear the same makeup *ALL THE TIME*, I always like to bring other stuff just in case I want to switch it up. Guess what, I never do. So to stop my packrat ways, I realized that the only thing I ever really change is my lipstick and MAYBE the eyeliner. SO I have a sleek little pouch with the following:

- Clean contact lens case filled with my tinted moisturizer on one side and primer/luminizer on the other

- MAC Mineralize Skinfinish powder

- Guerlain bronzer

- Hocus Pocus shadow

- eyebrow pencil

- Mascara

- A grey eyeliner (goes with more stuff)

- 3 lip-glosses (nude, pink, red).

I have ANOTHER smaller pouch with a roller ball fragrance, eye drops, travel size Yes to Cucumber wipes, hand sanitizer lip balm, NARS multiple stick (because I don't wear makeup on the plane but I want to put something on my face to wake it up when I arrive).

Liquids & gels. Security constraints now dictate how much we can take on the plane. So I simplified that as well. I use zip lock Baggies. If you pack them well, then you will always be ready to go when you travel. One has skincare items, which are all travel sized or blister packs. What I don't have in sample sizes, I put into small travel containers. The next one has body care (lotion, body oil, toothbrush, body wash, deodorant q-tips etc.). The last one has hair stuff again small samples of anti frizz, hair spray, elastics, Bumble styling cream, downy wrinkle release (which makes clothes smell awesome AND gets rid of wrinkles at the same time)

So even if you are a SERIOUS over-packer like me, you can be reformed!! I was and I never looked back!

17 MAKEUP AND YOUR TEENAGER ✔

I am going to share with you the most foolproof way to ensure that your daughter ends up looking like a rose and not a thorn when she starts wearing makeup. When she starts asking about when she can wear makeup, there are a few things you can do.

Establish a routine ahead of time. *Get her some skincare before you do anything.* It doesn't have to be expensive. In fact it's better if it isn't. She just needs to start using something to establish a routine. Explain to her that if she doesn't take care of her skin first, it won't matter what she puts on top of it.

Teach. After you have her using a regimen daily, buy her this *wonderful book* called, **Bobbi Brown Teenage Beauty**. Make a deal with her. Tell her to *read the book cover to cover and practice at home for 6 months* prior to her 16th birthday. Have her use some drugstore makeup (no makeup outside the house either). After she does that, tell her you will take her shopping for the good stuff. The book has valuable tips on taking care of your skin and makeup application that she will really benefit from.

Gift. After she has kept up her end of the bargain, make an appointment with the local Bobbi Brown counter in your area for her birthday and get her a gift card as a present. Tell the artist that she has read the book and has been practicing at home. Let your daughter work with the artist and stay within the parameters of the gift card that you have given her. She will also gain valuable skills from the artist as well. She will learn about using brushes, what brush goes with a certain makeup, how to blend and application techniques.

For your daughter's daily routine, it shouldn't be any more than the following:

1. Tinted moisturizer

2. Mascara

3. A little eyeliner

4. Blush/bronzer

5. Lip-gloss

When you give her those guidelines, she will learn how to interact with the artist, which is important. The great thing about Bobbi Brown makeup is that it is really hard to end up looking overdone. This way you both get what you want.

My friend Carrie did this for her twin girls and they totally appreciate and take care of the makeup (they are 19 or 20 now) – the point is, they established good habits early on. Not to mention they always look gorgeous, polished and pretty.

18 TOOLS 101 ✔

My first makeup kit was just thrown together. I was 17 and still working as a model in St. Louis while I finished high school. I was working at this store in the trendy Central West End neighborhood called *Barone.* It was the Eighties and makeup was CRAZY. Crazy colors, crazy textures you name it. Glitter everywhere!! From that job, I got to experiment and got my first set of professional brushes. As I honed my makeup artistry skills, I was also taught how to take care of them.

Brushes are definitely an investment and if you take care of them they will last you a good long time. There are definitely some brushes that are my favorites; Royal Crown, Sigma and MAC are a few brands that come to mind.

Here are a few tips to keep them clean. When using the wash method, make sure to take care and not submerge the *ferrule, which is the metal tube,* designed to hold the glued hair into place as well as providing a connection for the handle and the bristles. Soaking the brushes past the ferrule will loosen the glue. You should deep clean brushes once a month or more often depending on how often you use them.

Baby shampoo. This is one of the best ways to deep clean your brushes. Use one capful and a small amount of warm water in a cup or a jar. BE CAREFUL not to raise the water level above the bristles. Swish in the solution and leave to soak for 15 minutes. Rinse and let air dry.

Cinema secrets. This is a professional brush cleaner that is available for purchase online. It is known in makeup artist circles worldwide as one of the most effective cleansers. This is bright blue and has a vanilla scent. This is a quick-drying formula that cleans and sanitizes. It is safe for use with natural and synthetic hairs too. It immediately dissolves all traces of wax, liquid, and powder residue from brushes. Pour a small amount in a container and dip the brush in, swirl it around and remove. Wipe it clean on a tissue and let air dry for 2-5 minutes.

Anti-bacterial wipes. Makeup artist Billy B taught me this tip. These are a lifesaver, and a great way to clean your brushes in between deep cleans. Just swish your brush on the wipe until you don't see any residue of makeup.

Bar Soap. A bar soap like Dove has moisturizing properties so not only will it get your brush clean, but it will condition it as well. Wet your bar soap and rub your brush directly onto it. You can also massage the bristles to really work the soap in. Rinse until the water runs clear.

Olive Oil. For those hard to clean brushes that you use for gel liner, foundation and any other creamy substance. Remember oil dissolves oil. You can dip your brushes into a small bowl of olive oil to loosen any product buildup. Then follow with one of the soapy cleansing methods.

When using a soap method, always rinse your brushes until the water runs clear and lay them flat to dry on a towel. If you take care of your brushes, they will take care of you. I have read SO many online forums about how people just don't clean their brushes. It's not that difficult. If you don't clean them, you are opening yourself up to bacteria and your application will be muddy looking. So clean it up!

19 HAIR APPARENT ✔

Hair is always such a personal thing. Long, short, curly, straight. We all have issues and we all want it to look great. I learned a long time ago the best thing you can do for yourself is a *good haircut*.

When I was in 4th grade, I decided for some reason that I really wanted a haircut from a famous Olympian. All the other girls had it! It was dubbed the ***Dorothy Hamill Short & Sassy*** (she even had a shampoo & conditioner!). It was a wedge cut that the figure skater made famous at the 1976 Olympics. Problem was, I was a little black girl with curly hair. I begged my mother and she finally gave in and let me cut my hair, which by the way was well past my shoulders.

We went to the mall and I told the girl that I wanted a short and sassy like my friends. She looked at me and said, "Well, the best cut for YOUR hair is the shag". I said, "Okay, sure" not really knowing what that was. When she was done, I HATED IT. It was nothing like the "short and sassy" and to make matters worse; because my hair was curly it always looked shorter than it really was. I looked like a damn poodle.

The moral of that story is, ALWAYS pay good money for a

haircut, and stay out of the mall when you get it. Here are a few tips for all hair types to keep your hair looking great.

Deep condition. Do this once a week. This REALLY helps if you use a lot of hot tools on your hair.

Make your own protein treatment. This is great for all hair types. Mash an avocado and a banana together and pile the mixture onto your hair. Wrap in a plastic shower cap and place hot towel on top of that (just run a towel under HOT water and squeeze it out). You can also use mayonnaise for the same results. Leave on for 20 minutes, shampoo & condition as usual.

Rinse with apple cider vinegar. If you have a lot of buildup from styling products, you can pour a solution made from one cup of apple cider vinegar and one cup of water onto your hair. Whatever the shampoo didn't get...this will.

Always rinse with cool water. This always makes people cringe when I suggest it.... but it works. It closes the cuticle of the hair and makes it really shiny. I invested in a showerhead with an attachment so I can rinse my hair and not my whole body with the cool water.

Rinse with beer. This is another weird one that works for volume. Back in the 70's there was a shampoo/conditioner called *Body on Tap* that was made with ingredients from beer. The hops from the beer give you body and a whole lot of shine. Now not just any beer, you want a really yeasty hoppy one (an IPA will do). Let it sit until it reaches room temperature, shampoo your hair and squeeze out the excess water, then pour it on top. Let the beer sit for 5 minutes then rinse. Follow with your conditioner and voila shiny volumized hair.

Lemon juice for natural highlights. Yes it really works. Juice enough lemons to make 1 cup of juice and add to a bowl. Dilute that by adding an equal amount of water. If you are on the dry side add some leave in conditioner like infusium 21. Transfer to a spray bottle and spray on the areas you want to highlight. For more precise application you can use a cotton ball and select strands of hair. Make sure you condition your hair well because lemon juice can be drying.

Skip the hot tools. let your hair rest for the summer, or at least a few days. Let your hair air-dry.

Get an ionic dryer. if your hair is too thick to let dry naturally, invest in an ionic dryer to cut the drying time in half. Less heat on your hair cuts down on damage and gets you out the door faster.

EPILOGUE

I hope you enjoyed reading this book as much as I liked writing it. Sometimes it's fun to walk down memory lane and remember where you got your inspiration from in the first place. The women in my life, my mother, grandmothers and my sister have all inspired me in my beauty life in one form or another. I was practicing beauty looks on my sister when I was 8. We would get the hair magazines that had the diagrams of which way you should roll your hair to get the desired look. I was rolling hair, honey!

In 1976, we moved to St. Louis County. That was a big adjustment for us. We didn't fit in right away primarily because of the way we dressed. We were from California and our clothes were sorely out of place in the Midwest. We wore culottes and had knee high leather boots. I remember coming home and asking my mother for Levis and a down jacket after the first day.

Another thing that changed was the way my hair reacted to the environment. California is dry whereas the Midwest is extremely HUMID. My hair was a constant source of pain and humiliation (it sucked all of the moisture out of the air from May to September!) that is until I discovered products!

I tried them on myself and any of my friends that would let me near them. I would even typically cut friends hair at parties in high school (sometimes not that well but it still looked good!). I styled my friend Susan's hair in the bathroom regularly with my holy grail *Sebastian Shpritz Forte* (it was the 80's we ALL used that stuff). Looking back on that now, I'm kind of surprised that I didn't become a hairdresser. It was just a stone on my path, a part of my inspiration portrait. I thought that I wanted to be in fashion too. I styled all my friends and put together my "look" during high school. I was even voted best dressed in the high school superlatives, which was thrilling for a small county in the Midwest.

When it was time for college, I only wanted to go one place (and I only applied to one). I got accepted at Parsons School of Design in New York for the newly minted Fashion Merchandising program. I was SO EXCITED. I loved every second of it, especially being in New York in the late 80's. It was so alive with culture, art and excitement. Fashion was also another stone on my path, as that career was not meant to be for me.

I studied color theory (which helped me with custom blending for cosmetics) and fashion journalism (which helped me become a better writer). Taking and enjoying those courses made me question the path that I was on. I don't think I really realized it until I got a job at Bloomingdales. I worked for Borghese, they had a skincare line called Terme di Montecatini that was AMAZING and I still use the fango mud to this day. They sent me to school to learn about the products I was selling and I was DONE.... totally hooked. This is what I had been looking for! I went on to work for Lancôme, Clarins and finally becoming a custom blender for Prescriptives before hanging up my retail hat.

After spending a few passionless years in the corporate world working for Internet companies, I realized something was missing. I decided to pursue makeup artistry full-time. Soon I had a growing bridal artistry business that I enjoyed, but my heart wasn't in it. Something else was calling me. One day, one of my clients said to me, *"You know so much about everything, why don't you start a blog?"* "What's a blog?", I said. Never one to sit on the sidelines, I researched it, and started my own site. That site later became TheMakeupGirl.net. I have met many, many wonderful women that I now consider my friends and mentors after I started this journey. It was great to find others out there that were just like me.

You can ask anyone that has known me over my lifetime and they will tell you. I am always offering to pluck eyebrows, fill them in, give you a smokey eye or help you try out a new lipstick. It's just in my blood. Helping others is the cornerstone of any personal care profession. I like to think that I help others. It makes me feel good to do that. So I hope that I have helped you, even if it's just a little bit.

So even though beauty has always been my passion, it just took me a while to redirect myself back to it.

"Nearly every glamorous, wealthy, successful career woman you might envy now started out as some kind of schlepp."

– Helen Gurley Brown, Editor of Cosmopolitan Magazine

ABOUT THE AUTHOR

Lianne Farbes is passionate about educating consumers about beauty products. Her award wining blog TheMakeupGirl.net was voted best of the web by InStyle Magazine in 2009 and on of the top 50 beauty blogs by About.com and Konnector.com. She has leveraged her strengths and for the past 4 years she has organized a bi-annual sponsored event called Cocktails and Couture aimed at educating up and coming bloggers on the art of networking and honing your craft. For more information visit www.about.me/liannefarbes. You can follow Lianne on twitter at www.twitter.com/liannefarbes or at www.twitter.com/themakeupgirl